Foot yoga

A Guide to Happy, Healthy Feet

Becky Watson, E-RYT 200, RYT 500, PRYT, C-IAYT

©Copyright 2021 by Becky Watson-All rights reserved

"This is a wonderful day. I've never seen this one before."

–Maya Angelou

Contents

Before we begin.... 4
Chapter 1: Why Foot Yoga? 6
Chapter 2: Self-care starts with your feet 8
Chapter 3: How I came to learn about foot yoga 10
Chapter 4: Your foot needs to exercise too 13
Chapter 5: Step 1- Stretch Your Feet 16
    Toe Stretches 18
    Calf Stretch 24
    Curl the toes under 30
Chapter 6: Step 2 - Strengthen Your Feet................................. 33
    Toe Lifts... 36
chapter 7: Bonus tips 41
    Massage your feet 41
    Spread Those Toes! 43
    Use a Massage Ball 45
    Try a foot bath 47
    Practice Mindfulness... 48
Chapter 8: Conclusion... 50
A few things before you go.. 52

BEFORE WE BEGIN...

Congratulations! You've taken the first step towards healthier, happier feet. I'm so excited for you and I can't wait to hear how your feet feel after a little time with the exercises in this book.

I want to start right off and say that I'm not a foot doctor. What I've written here comes from years of working with people over the course of thousands of yoga classes. I've spent time observing my many yoga students and I've learned some tips and tricks that help your feet feel better. I'm grateful to be able to share what I know and it's my desire that you find a few ways to help your feet feel better in these pages.

With that said, what follows are some easy and practical tips that you can use to help your feet feel and function like they haven't in a long time. And...when your feet feel better, the rest of your body feels better too. It simply takes a few minutes out of your day for happier, healthier feet.

Disclaimer

This book is not intended to provide medical advice. As I stated above, I am not a doctor and do not provide medical advice. The contents of this book are for instructional purposes only. Always consult your medical practitioner before starting any fitness/exercise program or changing your habits. The contents of this book are not intended to be a substitute for a medical exam or medical advice.

CHAPTER 1: WHY FOOT YOGA?

The Merriam-Webster dictionary defines yoga as a system of physical postures, breathing techniques, and sometimes meditation These techniques are often practiced independently especially in Western cultures to promote physical and emotional well-being.

In my experience, yoga is so much more than putting your body in complex positions that look impossible at first. Yoga is also about your breath, your thoughts and how you feel in any given moment. It's about getting to know your body and it's also about noticing when something isn't working for your body. It's as much about awareness as it is about taking action to make a change.

Without awareness of what is happening right now, there can be no change. You must first notice what is happening right now before you can change to what you want.

This combination of awareness and change is what I've tried to put together in this book. My goal is to help you to become aware of what's happening in your feet so that you can begin to feel better.

Start by accepting that your feet ache or hurt sometimes and that this affects the rest of your body and mind. Next, accept that you can make a difference with your feet with a few changes in your daily routine. This awareness and change will take a little time and effort but the results will be worth it.

So, we're going to bring the practices of yoga to your feet. A little awareness mixed with some new ways of stretching and strengthening your feet.

Let's get started!

CHAPTER 2: SELF-CARE STARTS WITH YOUR FEET

How much do you think about your feet? I'm willing to bet that until they start hurting, you don't think too much about them. They get you where you need to go every day, support you as you stand around to work, cook, or chat, and they take you to fun places like the park or the beach.

Your feet are responsible for getting you from one place to another throughout the day, yet you don't spend too much time thinking about them or taking care of them. With all that your feet do for you, why not do something for them?

Now, I don't mean go and get a pedicure. Sure, having your toes freshly painted can make your feet look nice, but it doesn't do anything for the structure of your foot.

What about a massage or some foot exercises? What about soaking them in Epsom salts after a long day? There are so many actions that you can take to make your feet feel better and be healthier.

I've often heard that if your feet hurt, then the rest of your body hurts. Does that sound familiar to you?

Think back to a time when you spent too many hours on your feet. They were probably tired and/or aching. This led to the rest of you being tired and, most likely a bit cranky or out of sorts. Often something else in your body will hurt too.

Taking care of your feet can reverse this. After all, healthier feet feel better and will take you much farther in life. This book will outline several actions that you can take to create happier, healthier feet. Your feet will thank you for taking better care of them by feeling better than they have in a long time.

Once your feet feel better, then the rest of you will feel better too!

Are you ready to build stronger, healthier feet?

CHAPTER 3: HOW I CAME TO LEARN ABOUT FOOT YOGA

I've been teaching yoga for over 15 years. In the thousands of yoga classes that I have taught, I've seen a lot of feet. From healthy feet to feet that barely want to support a person. I've seen a wide variety of feet with high arches, no arches, bunions, hammer toes, misshapen toes, toes so squished together you can't separate them, and so on. All these feet have a story to tell about their owner, and if they could talk, your feet would tell your story, too.

Do you like your feet?

In a yoga class, we usually take our socks off. Right away, I can start to see how much care someone takes of their feet. If a student dislikes even looking at their feet, then this is often a sign that they have been neglecting their feet or that they are unhappy with their feet. I often hear comments about needing a pedicure just to make your feet presentable. Does that sound familiar?

Among many of my students and clients, there seems to be a common dislike of their feet. How about you?

> **Exercise:**
>
> Take a moment, right now, and just look at your feet. What do you notice? What do you like? What do you dislike? What do you feel in your feet? What do you feel about your feet? Just start with a visual examination of your feet & see where it takes you.

♦ ♦ ♦

Are your feet talking?

What's interesting to me is that when you neglect a part of your body, in this case, your feet, then that part of your body will start to talk to you in one form or another. If you don't listen to what your feet are saying, then that discussion will get louder and louder until you have no choice but to pay attention. Suddenly, it hurts to walk or even just stand and you are left with little choice but to do something that will help your feet.

You might be asking yourself...How did I get here?

So often, what happens is that you've developed a habit of mistreating your feet. You're constantly putting them into shoes that are too small or too narrow to allow them to form their natural state, for example. This can result in misshapen toes that just don't feel good. Or maybe you grip with your toes out of anxiety or habit, and this can contribute to having hammer toes. Putting too much pressure on one part of your foot can contribute to bunions. Not exercising or stretching the foot can lead to Plantar Fasciitis.

All these foot conditions can be painful if left untreated.

Over my years of teaching classes, I've learned several ways to work with feet so that they function and feel better. The simple exercises that I've included in this book have been given to countless people. Often, those same people have come back to me, sometimes months later, to say how much better their feet feel. These simple exercises were so helpful to them that they made a point to thank me.

This tells me that these exercises can work for other people too.

The exercises in this book are free and easy to do. Except for a couple, you don't even need any equipment. They are easy to practice and they work so well. While I won't promise that these exercises and tricks will fix all your foot problems, I will tell you that your feet can feel better. Of course, how much better depends on a lot of variables, but when your feet hurt, even feeling a little bit better is a blessing. And...when your feet feel better, then the rest of your body feels better.

So, why are you waiting? Take better care of your feet today!

CHAPTER 4: YOUR FOOT NEEDS TO EXERCISE TOO

There are over 100 muscles, ligaments, and tendons in a foot. There are also 33 joints. That's a lot of tissue in a small, compact space, and a lot of places where the foot can bend.

It's no wonder that when we consistently put our feet in shoes that don't fit well or are too small, that our amazing feet lose the ability to perform as they were designed to do.

These muscles, ligaments, and tendons need to be stretched just like other parts of your body, and all your joints will be a part of this. If you've ever spent any time stretching, then you know how good it can feel to do so. Well, the same can be said about stretching a foot. It'll feel good, and you'll wonder why you haven't done these stretches before.

Have you stretched your feet in a class before?

If you've ever been to an exercise class (yoga or any other type), then you've been taken through stretches for the body. These stretches are usually designed to increase flexibility and blood flow to the various parts of your body and to keep you from getting any injuries. In general, these stretches that you're doing keep your body healthier.

Now, think back to the last exercise class that you did. Were there any foot stretches? Did the instructor say anything about how to make your feet healthier? Chances are the answer to those questions is a "no." Usually, whether in a formal class, book, or video, the focus is on the larger muscles in the body. We stretch our arms, legs, backs, sides of the body, etc., but we tend to overlook the feet.

It's time to change that!

Before we go any further, it's time to do a self-assessment.

The first thing that you need to do is **take off your shoes**.

I know for some of us, that's a huge step. I know people who only take off their shoes to bathe or go to bed. They absolutely refuse to go barefoot for any length of time. This saddens me because wearing shoes constantly will slowly weaken the foot. The foot begins to rely on the shoe for support and the muscles will be used less than if you were barefoot. This can create a downward cycle where your feet become weaker from shoes and so you wear your shoes more often to protect your feet.

If this describes you, then I'm really challenging you from the beginning.

Now that your shoes are off, really look at your feet!

Start by just looking at your feet. Notice any changes that have happened over time. Do you have some bunions or hammer toes? Are your toes crowded from narrow shoes? Are your arches high or low? Do you even have visible arches in your feet?

Practice a little awareness now to give yourself a good baseline of what your feet are like. Maybe even take a picture so that you don't have to rely on your memory. That way, when you look at them in a week, month, or year, you'll notice any changes that you see.

How well do your feet move right now?

A foot can move in multiple ways. I like to think that they are remarkable feats of engineering. Let's explore just a bit.

Spend a moment just wiggling your toes, pointing and flexing your feet, turning them from side to side. Notice the various ways that your feet can naturally move. Also, notice any ways in which your movement is limited. Take this time to really get to know how your feet can move right now.

After you've practiced the exercises in this book for a while, then come back to this same self-assessment and notice any changes in your feet.

Now, if you're finding that your range of movement is limited, then these stretches and exercises can help you to regain your mobility. It just takes a little time and patience. So, let's get started...

CHAPTER 5: STEP 1- STRETCH YOUR FEET

We're starting with foot stretches because pretty much everyone that I meet has tightness in their feet and ankles. Just taking time to stretch even once or twice a week will help to eliminate this tightness.

In this chapter, you'll find stretches for your toes & bottom of your feet, calf stretches and ankle stretches. Try them all at least once. Then pick which ones you need the most and continue to practice them. If you find that you need all of the stretches, don't worry. It's common and I see that a lot!

Props will be helpful.

For some of these stretches, it really does help to have something to prop your toes on. I like to use a yoga block, but a corner of a wall can work as well. If you prefer a yoga block, then you can often find one for less than $10. My favorite places to get yoga blocks are Target or TJ Maxx but since yoga has become so popular, you can find them all over the place. I've even seen them at pharmacies lately. You don't need to spend a lot of money on a yoga block. I've yet to find one that doesn't work well.

However, if you don't want to purchase a yoga block, then using the wall or something like a yoga block is just fine. I like to be creative & use whatever props are handy. I encourage you to do the same. For these stretches a corner of a wall will work just as well as a yoga block.

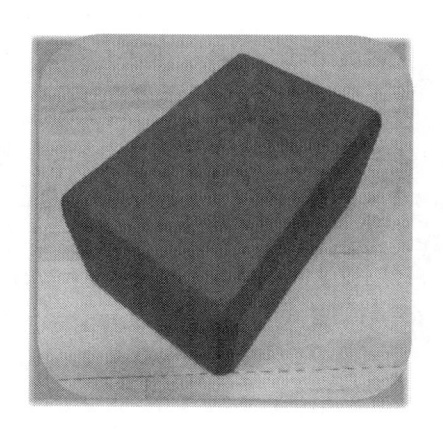

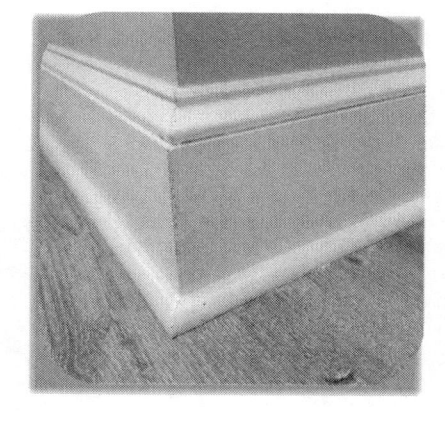

Yoga Block

Corner of a wall

TOE STRETCHES

I use these toe stretches in yoga classes frequently, and my yoga students love it! There are three main variations of these toe stretches. Try them all to see what works best for your own feet. You probably need all these stretches, but you'll benefit from doing just one of them.

Before you do though, check out your balance first.

I suggest that you practice your balance before you begin to stretch your toes. Why? Because when your feet are tight, it's harder to balance. Starting here will help illustrate to you just how much you can benefit from stretching out those feet. After you've done the exercises in this book, do the same balance exercise. If you're like most of my students and clients, you'll find that your balance is better after stretching your feet.

> **Exercise:**
>
> **For this balance pose (from a standing position), simply lift up one foot. It doesn't have to be lifted up very high. Just lift your foot off of the floor. Then close your eyes. Notice your balance and when you're ready, switch sides and try it on the other foot. Once you've done that, then you are ready to move on to the stretches below.**

Toe Stretch 1

For the first foot stretch, place all of the toes of your right foot on a block or wall and let the foot slide down the block. Hold this position for about a minute.

If you've never stretched your foot, that minute might feel like a lifetime, but stay with it. It really doesn't take a long hold to begin to change your foot. A minute is plenty of time to begin to stretch that connective tissue in your foot.

After that minute wiggle your toes just a bit before you move on to the next stretch.

I've included some pictures that illustrate doing this stretch with a yoga block and also using the corner of a wall.

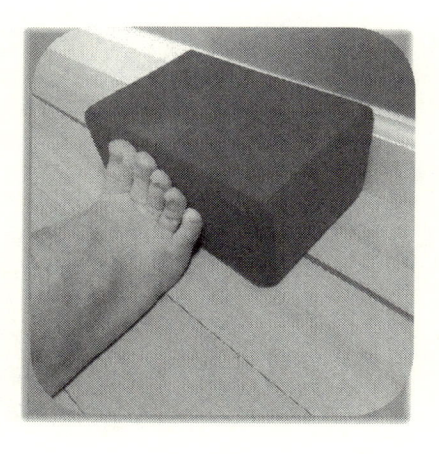

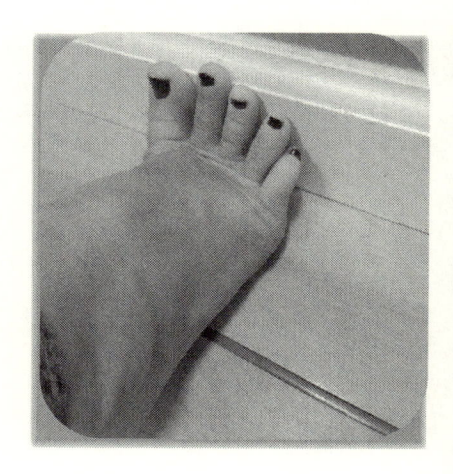

Toe Stretch 2

For the second one, you'll go over to the right corner of the same block (or find a position on a wall where you can do this). Place your big toe on the block and let the other four toes go down to the floor. Again, you only need to hold this for about a minute. That minute may seem like a short time, but it's enough to begin to have healthier feet.

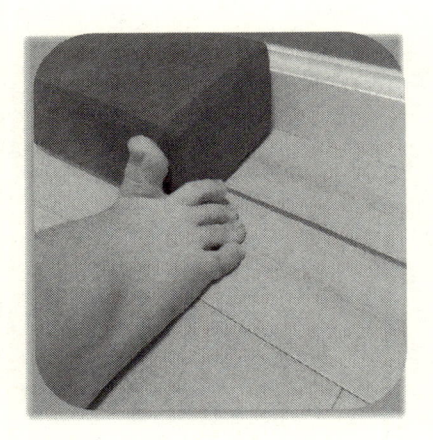

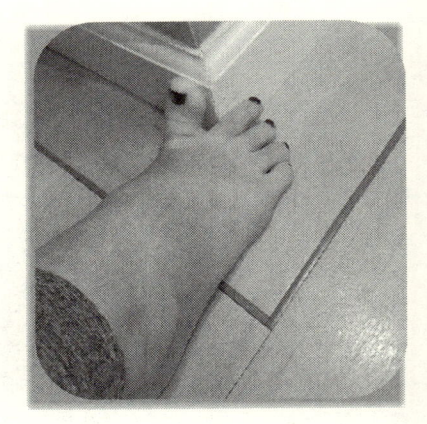

Toe Stretch 3

For the third stretch, go over to the left corner of the block and place your four toes on the block and let the big toe go down to the floor. Now, I've found that with many people, the big toe won't easily go down to the floor. If that is happening for you, then you can use the other foot to encourage the toe down to the floor. Yes, I do mean to step on it and push it down, gently, of course. Again, hold for about a minute.

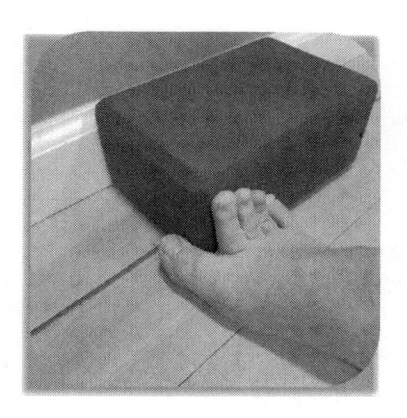

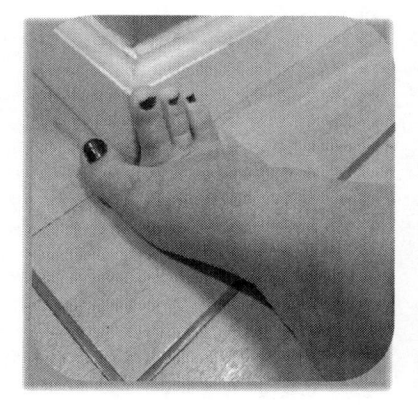

Pause and notice.

Now, after you have completed these toe stretches on the right foot, pause to place both feet flat on the floor. Notice the difference in your feet.

I always feel like my foot is much more awake after doing these stretches, and it's obvious when I have done one foot and not the other one. After comparing your feet, repeat the above 3 stretches for your left foot. You'll do all the toes, move to the left corner of the block, and have the big toe up and the other toes down, and then move to the right corner of the block so that the four toes are on the block and the big toe is down on the floor.

> **Exercise:**
>
> **Now that you've stretched both feet, go back to that balance pose that I had you do first. Simply life one foot and close your eyes. Try it on both sides. Notice your balance. Has it improved?**

For most people that I've worked with in a yoga class, the answer to whether your balance is better is a definite yes. Your feet can function so much better just by adding in some simple stretches. It will take you maybe 10 minutes to do all of these toe stretches as well as the balance pose before and after the stretches.

It's a worthy investment of your time!

What would it be like to have your feet feel better? Is it worth 10 minutes a couple of times a week to change your feet?

I think that investing time in your feet to help them feel better is a smart investment, and you will too once you begin to take more care of your feet.

This is the main exercise that helps my students and clients.

These simple stretches are the basis of what I've given to countless people in my yoga classes over the years. This is what has had so many people come back to me weeks or even months later and make a point of saying how much better their feet feel. Occasionally, I'll give them a few other pointers on things that they can do for their feet. However, most of the people that I teach get just these stretches and walk away happier with their feet than they've been in a long time.

You can stop here and just do these few stretches and you'll begin to feel better. However, if you'd like to take your foot health even further, then read on to get some more tips and ideas for the healthiest feet that you've had in a long time. I know that you'll be glad that you did!

CALF STRETCH

I've found that stretching your calf helps your foot feel better. Why is that? It's because the soft tissue of your body is not isolated. It's connected to surrounding tissue as well. So, when you want to work on the health of your feet, move up your leg a bit and stretch your ankles and calves as well.

With this calf stretch, you'll not only be stretching your calf but also the soft tissue in your ankle and your Achilles tendon as well.

This is one of my favorite stretches lately. I find that my feet and legs feel better when I take the time to stretch out my calves. That's because I naturally point my feet more than flex my ankles. This causes my calf muscles to be tighter. So, with this stretch, I'm relieving some of that tightness.

The stretch that I'm including here is one that I came across accidentally one day. I rested my foot partly on a sandbag with my heel on the floor. I played around with the placement a bit and I immediately felt the stretch in my calf.

Since that day, I've used this stretch with clients and students and they all tell me how much better their legs feel.

Now it's your turn!

Here's how to do these calf stretches.

You'll need a prop for this one. I like to use a sandbag that I have in my office, but I've also used a yoga block. You could also use any other firm surface that is stable and will lift your foot off the floor a couple of inches.

I like to take the prop (sandbag, block, or another firm surface) and place it against the base of a wall. You can stabilize the prop by placing it against the wall and then you'll be able to also use the wall for support and balance.

Check out the pictures on the next few pages to better understand your foot placement.

Version 1

Once you've got the prop in place, then you'll start by placing about half of your foot up on the prop. Leave your heel down on the floor. Make sure that your foot is pointing straight ahead for this one. Now you can lean forward toward the wall to increase the stretch or away from the wall to decrease the stretch. Hold the stretch for a minute before releasing the foot.

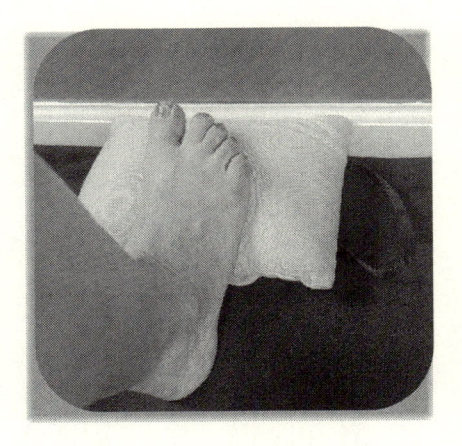

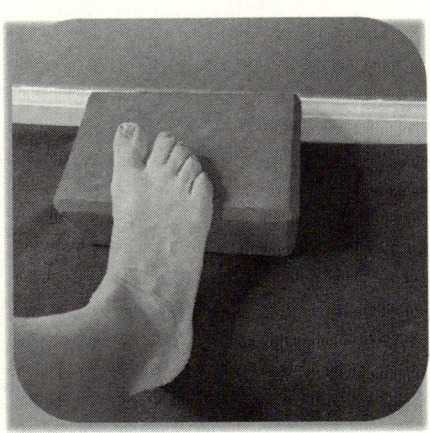

Version 2

For this second version, again start with about half of your foot on your prop but turn your toes out as much or as little as you want. Play with it a bit & discover how far feels right. Make sure that your heel is still down on the floor. Again, you can lean into the wall or away from the wall to get the intensity of the stretch that you want. Hold the stretch for a minute before releasing your foot.

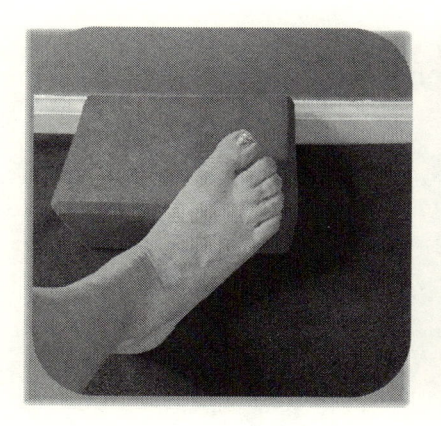

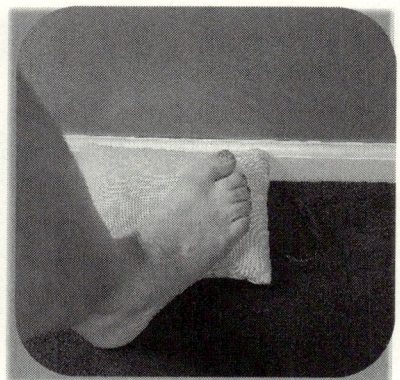

Version 3

For this last version, start with about half of your foot on the prop & then turn your toes in. How much or how little depends on how much stretch you need or want. With your heel down on the floor, lean toward the wall or away from the wall to increase or decrease the intensity. Hold this version for a minute as well.

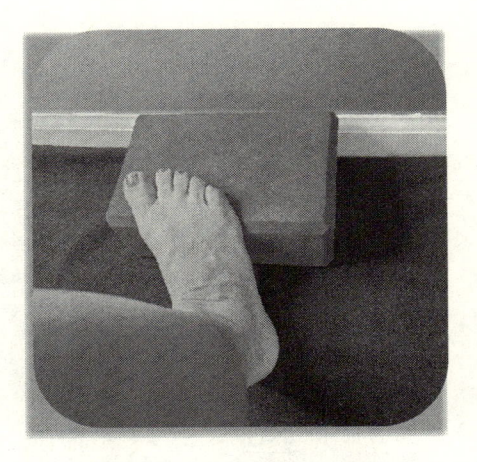

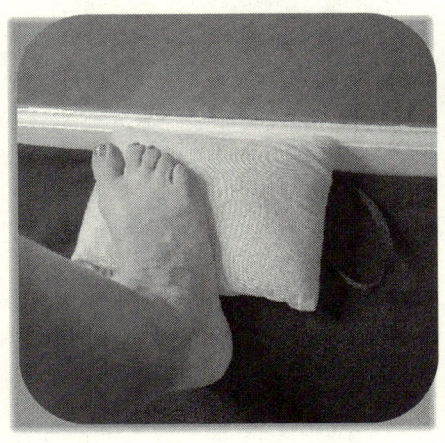

♦ ♦ ♦

When you've done all three versions on one foot, pause. Place both feet flat on the floor. Notice any differences in your feet and legs. Then move over to the other foot and give it some love as well.

CURL THE TOES UNDER

After you've stretched out the back of the ankle and the calf muscle, you'll want to stretch the opposite side of the ankle & the front of the foot. This will help with your overall flexibility and mobility.

I have two slightly different versions of this stretch for you. You'll want to try them both. You'll find illustrations on the following couple of pages.

When you've done both versions of this stretch on the right foot, pause, and place both feet on the floor. Again, notice any differences in your feet, ankles and legs and then move over to the left foot.

Version 1

Start with the right foot. From a standing position, simply curl all the toes of the right foot under. Don't put a lot of your weight on that right foot. Just curl the toes under & allow them to stretch a bit. If you're balance challenged like a lot of my clients, you might want to do this stretch near a wall so that you can place a hand on the wall for a little bit of support. Working on your balance is a bonus for this exercise! Hold the stretch for a minute then move on.

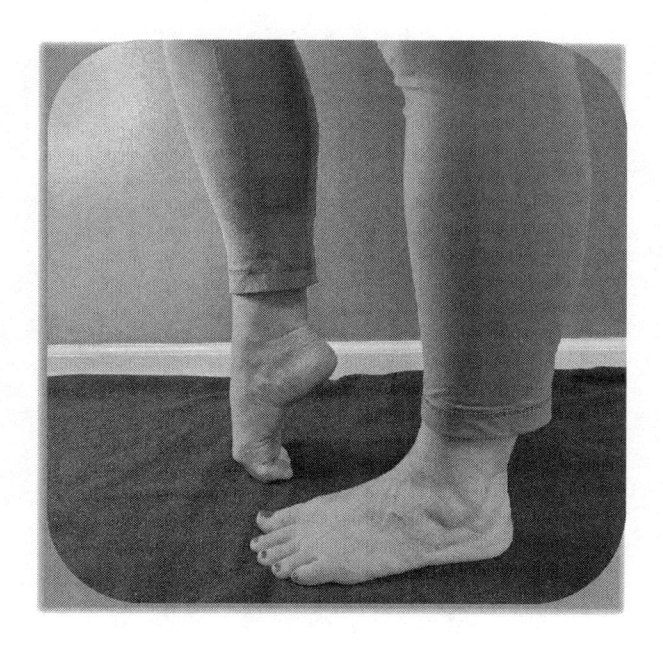

Version 2

For the second version, keep your toes curled under and step your right foot back as far as you'd like. You'll be shifting the stretch and likely feel it on the top of your foot and maybe in the ankle as well. Use the wall for support if you need it. Again, hold the stretch for a minute.

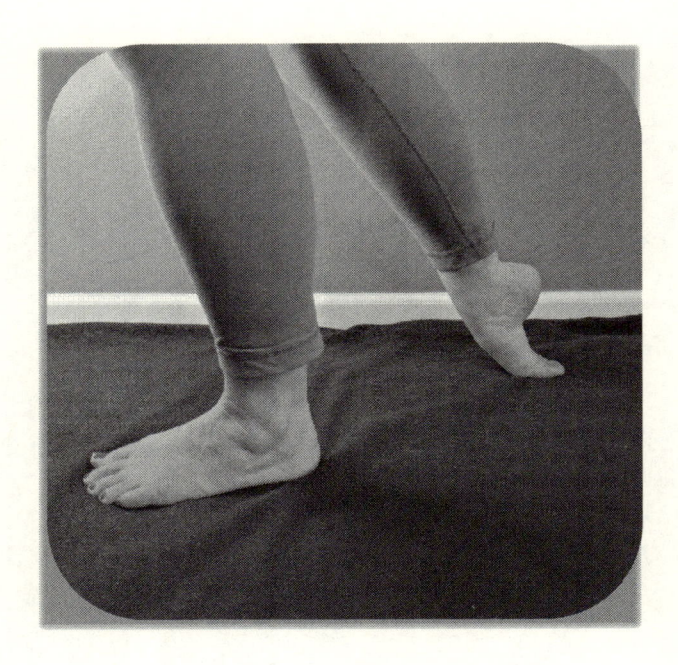

CHAPTER 6: STEP 2 - STRENGTHEN YOUR FEET

When you think of stretching a muscle, the opposite of that would be strengthening, right? Well, I have a few simple strengthening exercises that you can do with your feet as well.

My first suggestion is simple.

Go barefoot.

Of course, one of the best things you can do for your feet is to simply go barefoot. When you are barefoot, all parts of the foot are being used. When you stand barefoot, your weight will be more evenly distributed. If it's not, then you will quickly notice if you are leaning to the side and placing more of your weight on one part of the foot. You will automatically shift to balance and have a more even distribution of your weight.

When you have shoes on, it's not so obvious that you're placing more emphasis on the inner or outer part of your foot. A shoe will mask this because of the cushion that is built into the shoe. So, take off those shoes for a few minutes each day.

Many people have spent so much of their lives in shoes, that the thought of being barefoot is foreign to them. It might even be painful because your foot has gotten so weak. So, my suggestion is to just begin with small amounts of time. If you're someone who rarely goes barefoot, then start by just waiting 10 or 15 minutes after you shower to put shoes back on. Or maybe when you first come home, instead of changing into comfy slippers, walk around barefoot for a few minutes.

No matter how you fit this into your day, start small. Your feet will be weak and not used to the extra work that being barefoot will require of them. The good news is that even short amounts of time being barefoot will strengthen your feet. Over time, increase the amount of time that you are barefoot and start to notice how different your feet feel.

Feet really were designed to be barefoot. I like to think of them as masterpieces of design. You can move them in so many different ways, but over time with shoes on, we tend to lose some of that functionality. Going barefoot more often will begin to bring back some of the lost mobility into your feet.

I know that most people don't have jobs where they can stand around barefoot. Being a yoga teacher does have its perks sometimes! I also realize that it's not practical to ask you to spend all day barefoot. What I am asking is that you kick off your shoes while you're at home a little more often. Give those feet a chance to breathe and move. Let those toes wiggle. Feel the freedom that goes with being barefoot. Try it and see how it feels!

> **Exercise:**
>
> Take off your shoes and walk around for a few minutes. Notice your feet as you do so. How does it feel to have those feet come into direct contact with the ground? How do your feet feel with each step? Does it hurt to walk barefoot? Is one foot more flexible than the other? Do your toes flex as you walk or are they stiff?

Try not to judge your feet or yourself for how those feet feel. Just be aware of how they are in this moment so that you know what you need/want to change about your feet.

TOE LIFTS

Sometimes your feet are achy because they've spent so much time in shoes that they've actually become weaker. When your feet are being supported by shoes, they don't have to work as hard to adjust to the various surfaces that they would encounter if you were barefoot. Because of this, the muscles of the feet can weaken and ache. If you're noticing how much your feet ache, it's a clue that your feet are sending to you. Listen to your feet.

So, when I've had people asking how to make their feet healthier, I've often given them some foot exercises to do. Again, these same people come back and tell me how much better their feet feel.

These toe exercises are fairly easy to do. They just take a little time out of your day and you can do them just about anywhere. You can also do them from a seated or standing position.

So, no excuses. Try these toe exercises!

There are a couple of different versions that I'll introduce to you. Basically, these are exercises for your toes. Just like you can do exercises for your arms to make them stronger, you can also do exercises for your toes that will make your feet feel better.

Here are the different variations for you to try. I suggest working with one foot at a time, but if you're feeling advanced today, you can do both of your feet at the same time.

Version 1

Let's start with the right foot. Stand or sit with your right foot flat on the floor. No shoes and no socks.

Now lift just your big toe up off the floor. You want to keep the rest of the foot on the floor. I'm going to guess that you're not used to lifting just one toe at a time. Be patient. Let your foot figure out how to move in this manner. It will get easier with practice!

Repeat this toe lift for 10-20 times. You'll begin to feel it in the arch of your foot and maybe even further up your leg. That's okay. You're using your muscles a bit differently and they'll grow stronger as you practice this more often.

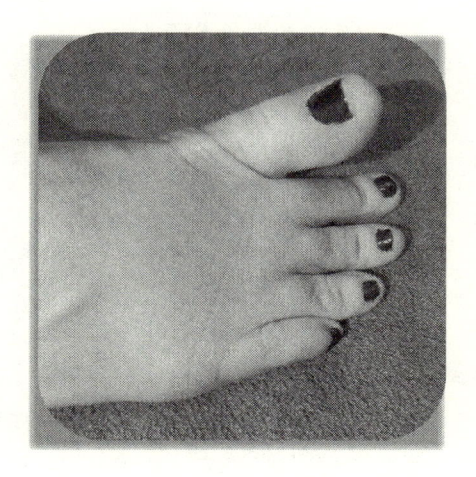

Lift just that big toe.

Version 2

Now for this second version, you're going to reverse the action. You'll keep the big toe down and lift the other four toes off of the floor.

This might be even weirder for you to try. You might even need some help to do this movement. If you do need help, that's okay. You can use one of your hands to hold down the big toe while you lift the rest of the toes up. The rest of the foot stays on the floor.

Again, do this 10-20 times for each foot. With time, it will get easier & you'll be able to do it without your hands holding the big toe down.

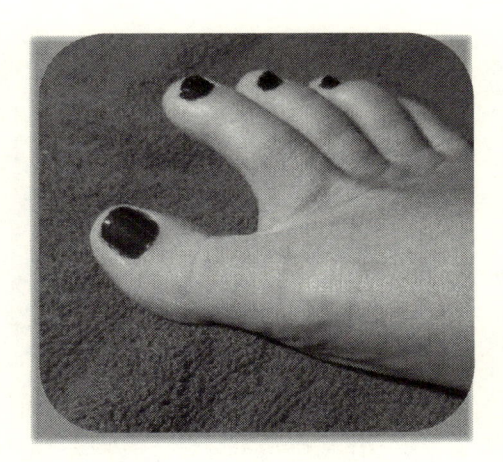

Keep that big toe down & lift the other four toes.

Version 3

I usually call this version the bonus round. When you can do this round without using your hands to hold down your toes, then you know that your feet are getting stronger! Don't worry though. If you're still using your hands to help your feet with this stretch, then your foot is still working hard at getting stronger.

For this final version, you'll keep your big toe down and your pinky toe down while you lift the 3 toes in the middle.

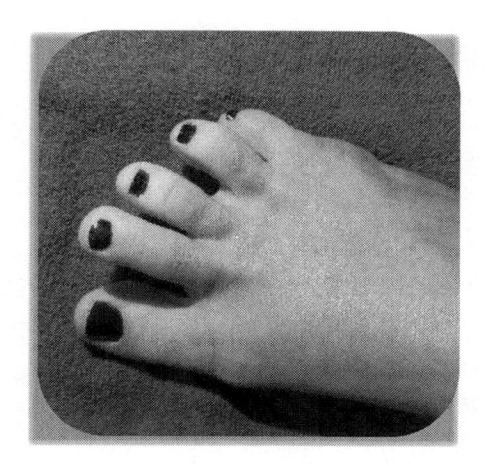

Keep your big toe & little toe down.

Most people I show this to think that I'm a little bit crazy. You probably think that right now too and that's ok with me. I know that these toe lifts help your feet, and this bonus round version gives you the chance to improve your feet even more.

Again, you can also use your hand to hold down the big toe and pinky toe when you first start to practice this. While you're lifting those middle toes, do what you need to do to keep the rest of the foot on the floor. It's ok to cheat a little bit. Your feet aren't used to this type of activity, but with just a little bit of time and practice, your feet can get used to this movement and get stronger at the same time. Soon you won't even need to cheat at it!

Question:
How often do I need to practice these toe lifts?

You can do them daily. It's a gentle exercise that will just make your feet feel better over time.

If you find that your feet are stronger than you thought, then you might only need to do these a few times a week. Notice how your feet are feeling after the exercise. If your feet are a little tired after these exercises, then they've worked more than normal and you probably need to do these more often.

So, judge how often you need to do the exercises based on how your feet feel.

CHAPTER 7: BONUS TIPS

MASSAGE YOUR FEET

Most people love a good foot massage. It feels good for the feet and stimulates other parts of the body at the same time. You have a lot of acupressure points in your foot that connect to other parts of the body. So, a foot massage is like a massage for other parts of the body at the same time. Bonus!

Massaging your feet also helps to loosen the muscles and connective tissue in your feet. Some of those aches in your feet are caused by tight muscles or connective tissue. Taking a few minutes to rub your feet can bring a little relief to them.

Question:
How do I massage my feet?

There's really not a perfect way to massage your feet. So, don't worry about doing it wrong.

It can be nice to start with a favorite lotion or some massage oil in your hands. Then begin to rub your feet. Start with some lighter strokes and then, if it feels right, you can focus on any tight spots that you feel. You'll quickly get to know your feet this way. Maybe there's one spot that's always sore. If that's happening, then spend a little extra time on that spot. Be firm but gentle. Don't forget the top of the foot or the heel and ankle. Also, try pulling on the toes and wiggling them back and forth a bit.

No matter how you massage your feet, you'll be increasing the blood flow, relaxing and releasing the soft tissue of the foot and releasing stress throughout the body.

Go ahead and give it a try!

SPREAD THOSE TOES!

It can also feel nice to place a finger in between each toe. Try to work a finger in between each toe all at the same time.

While this isn't really a massage, after spending all day smooshed into shoes that are really constricting, this will most likely feel good. Whenever I practice this, I notice a release of tension further up my leg. Yes, releasing tension in your feet will help release it in other parts of your body. It's all connected!

Spread out your toes. Give your feet the space that they crave. If you're lucky enough to walk barefoot often, then your feet will naturally spread out a bit. By putting a finger between each toe, you're just helping those toes find a naturally spacious experience.

Do it often enough and your feet will start to feel better from not being forced into a shape that's not natural to them!

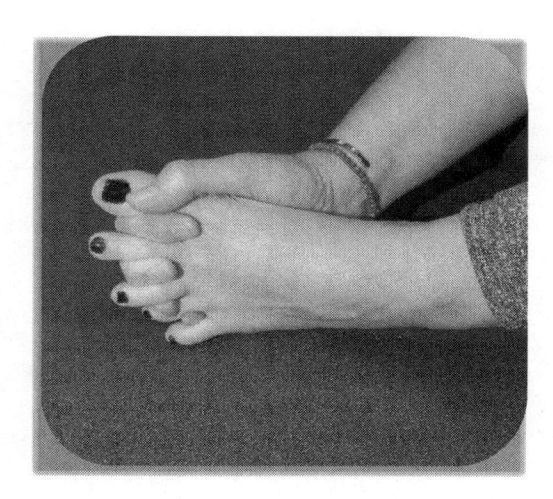

Place a finger between each toe

Another simple idea is to simply spread your toes apart. In the pictures below, you can see a foot with the toes as they normally are. The second picture shows the toes spread apart.

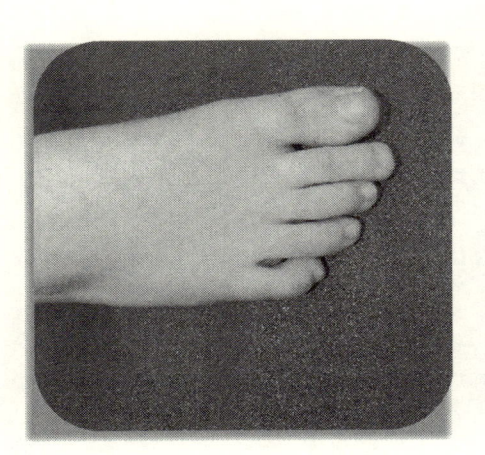

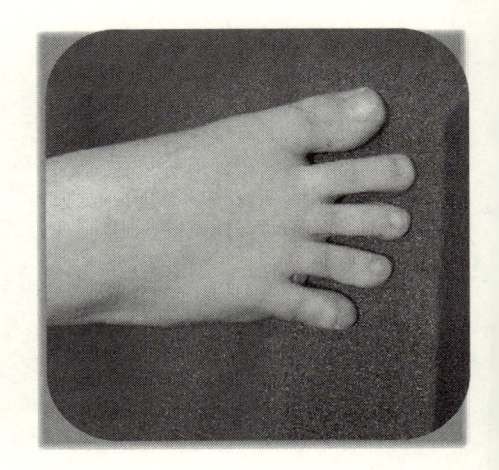

At first, this might be difficult to do, but the more you practice simply putting a little space between the toes, the easier it will be. Of course, the more you go barefoot, the more you'll be giving those toes a chance to spread naturally. You won't even have to think about it!

USE A MASSAGE BALL

My next suggestion is to try using a Massage Ball.

I have several small massage balls that I use with my clients and on my own feet. They're so helpful when you want to massage your feet and put a little extra emphasis on one spot.

I'll be honest... this might hurt a bit.

If you've got tight/sore spots, then this might be a bit more painful than if you massage your own feet. However, these massage balls do a terrific job of getting deeper into the tissue of the foot than you would with your own fingers.

How do you use a massage ball?

Well, there are multiple ways.

You can use your hand to move the ball around your foot and enjoy the massage. Simply move the ball around all over the top and the bottom of the foot. Don't forget the sides as well.

You can also take the ball and place it under your foot. Then, using a little of your body weight for extra pressure, you can begin to move your foot around on the ball. Again, this might hurt a bit because you're using extra pressure to go deeper into the tissue of the foot.

So, judge the pressure based on how deep you want to go. Remember less is often more! In this case that might mean that you use just a little of your body weight and that will be enough. Practice kindness to yourself. Don't do too much too fast. I want you to be able to walk comfortably after this foot massage.

TRY A FOOT BATH

A great way to relieve tired, stressed, or sore feet is a foot bath.

It's as simple as filling a small tub with warm water and adding in Epsom salts. You can also add in your favorite essential oil for added benefit. The Epsom salts will help to relieve soreness and swelling in the feet. They'll help to reduce your overall stress level. They'll also give you some extra magnesium and that magnesium will speed your recovery from standing on those feet all day long. It might even help you sleep better. There are so many benefits to using Epsom salt in your foot bath.

The essential oils can help your feet even more. I like a little **lavender oil** in my foot bath. The lavender helps to reduce inflammation and stress. It also helps to calm my mind and body at the same time for an overall sense of relaxation.

Some other suggested oils include...

Eucalyptus Oil can provide a cooling effect for your muscles as well as reduce pain and inflammation.

Peppermint Oil can revive tired feet.

Marjoram Oil can calm and soothes your muscles.

There are a lot of good options when it comes to essential oils. It might be that some days one oil is just what you need and other days, you need something else. Experiment and find the oils that work for you.

PRACTICE MINDFULNESS

How often do you pay attention to your feet?

Usually, you notice your feet when they hurt but ignore them the rest of the time. What if you practiced a little mindfulness around your feet?

Whenever you can, go barefoot and just notice what it feels like to walk around barefoot. Notice what it feels like to place your feet on the ground. Notice any sensations that move up your body from your feet. Notice if you have a preference for walking on one surface over another. Just begin to notice what happens when your feet touch the ground.

You can also practice mindfulness when you have shoes on. How do your feet feel in your shoes? Do your shoes encourage your foot to spread out a bit or are your shoes making your feet feel cramped? Do you need new shoes to make your feet feel better?

Again, notice how it feels to take a step in your shoes. Notice if your shoes are making your feet feel energized or if they're making you feel tired. Notice if the rest of your body feels good while in your shoes or if your shoes are leading you to not feel good throughout the day. Also, notice if you're placing style over function.

I won't tell you that you have to go and buy shoes that are ugly, but make your feet feel great. However, I will ask that you try mindfulness in your shoes. Be aware of how your feet and the rest of your body feel while you're wearing your shoes.

Maybe you want to stick with the pretty but uncomfortable shoes. That's okay! You can do that. Just be aware of how you feel while you wear those shoes.

CHAPTER 8: CONCLUSION

It's my hope that you've learned one or two things from this book about making your feet happier and healthier. It's my desire to help you have feet that feel better, because the better that your feet feel, then the better the rest of you will feel.

Try out a foot stretch or a foot strengthener. See how much better your feet can be. And, remember that it does take a little time for your feet to heal and feel better.

Your feet won't get stronger and become more flexible overnight. It probably took years for your feet to get to this uncomfortable stage, and it will take a little time to reverse this process. Be consistent and stick with it.

I've had so many people come back to me and say that these exercises have helped their feet. I know that they can be helpful for you as well. Give them a try, and feel better, sooner.

Finally, on a personal note, I've had my own bouts with plantar fasciitis. I've used the toe stretches and the toe lifts to help my own feet feel better. It doesn't take a lot of time out of my day, but it does take consistency. I know that when I've been neglecting my feet and they start to hurt, then it's time for me to stretch and strengthen them.

I'm like everyone else. I get busy and forget about all that my feet do for me. However, having a little plantar fasciitis in my feet is a great reminder for me to take time for my own self-care.

There's no better time than right now for you to join me in taking better care of your feet! Grab a yoga block or a massage ball or just go to the wall and begin today.

A FEW THINGS BEFORE YOU GO...

I would like to acknowledge all the many yoga students that I've had the pleasure to teach over the past 15+ years. Although I'm labeled your teacher in class, I know that I've learned just as much, if not more, from each of you. Every time that I step in front of a group of students, I'm honored to share what little I feel that I know about this time-honored tradition. Each day, each class is a chance to learn something new about myself. I continue to teach so that I can continue this exploration for both myself and for my students.

I want to acknowledge my son Alex who helped me originally put together this book. Without him, I'd probably still be trying to figure out how to format everything!

Also, thank you to Holly Howe for her continued support and unwavering confidence in all that I do!

If you liked this book, I would very much appreciate a review on Amazon. Your reviews can help lead other people to this information and then they too will have happier, healthier feet.

If you'd like to learn more about the yoga therapy that I practice, I can be found at beckywatsonyoga.com.

And remember...it's never too late to live happier & healthier!

May you laugh more,
May you rest more,
May you judge less,

Namaste

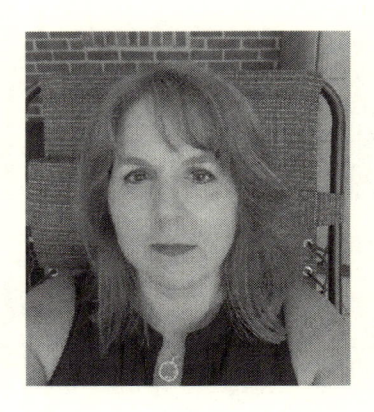

About the Author

Becky has been teaching yoga classes since 2006 and is now a IAYT certified yoga therapist. She loves to work with people who never thought that they could practice yoga.

Now, Becky helps women feel better physically, mentally, and emotionally by moving on from previous trauma and finding a yoga practice that supports them in living healthier and happier. She believes that it's never too late to start and that you must start right where you are to move forward in life. You'll feel a bit better with each step that you take.

When not teaching a class or leading a private therapy session, Becky can be found at home with her dog, Max. In her spare time, she likes to hike in the nearby mountains, pull a few weeds in her yard and read.

She can be reached at becky@beckywatsonyoga.com.

Made in the USA
Columbia, SC
05 December 2021